Table of Contents

The UK Keto Diet Book For Beginners 2021

Quick, Healthy and Delicious Recipes for the Whole Year incl. Meal Prep and Diet Plan

Amber W. Davies

ISBN- 9798592210709

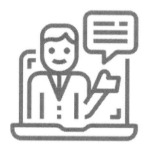

The Keto diet is a dietary regimen which focuses on food that can provide your body with a lot of healthy fats and proteins, reducing the amount of carbs. The goal is to get adequate calories and energy from fat rather than carbs.

If you want to try the keto diet, here you will find plenty of tips and a comprehensive overview of what you can eat. More importantly, we will show you a world full of delicious recipes you can easily make at home, even if you are not a professional chef, to enjoy everyday homemade and genuine food which will provide your body with plenty of healthy nutrients.

Losing weight and feeling better has never been easier!

The Keto Diet: A Guide for Beginners

The keto diet is particularly useful for losing weight, excess body fat, or reducing hunger. However, this alimentary regimen can also be the perfect starting point to switch to a healthier lifestyle, with plenty of genuine and homemade food. This diet has been rising in popularity over the last few years, with people from all around the world praising its benefits.

If you are curious to try the keto diet, you should first understand the basics. As it often happens with new alimentary regimens, at first it might be difficult to completely change your lifestyle. For this reason, understanding how to approach your new diet and what food you should eat to feel better is the best way to enjoy your food and never give up.

What Does "Keto" Mean

Keto, or ketogenic, refers to ketosis. This is a process in which your body produces specific molecules called ketones, which are used to give you energy. This works as an alternative fuel source whenever your blood sugar supply is low.

When you reduce your amount of carbs and calories, your liver starts producing ketones from fat. These are then used by all your body, including the brain, to help you get through your daily activities. This makes your entire body switch to a different fuel supply, which is run mostly on fat. This means that it is easier for your body to burn fat off, leading to a quicker and easier weight loss.

This can also have different benefits for your health, including less hunger, a steady supply of energy, and an improved skin appearance.

An alternative way to reach ketosis is by fasting, which is not eating anything. However, medical professionals do not recommend this practice, as our ketosis won't last forever and you won't be able to rely on a steady health condition.

What to Eat on A Ketogenic Diet?

Meat

The keto diet requires a high amount of fats rather than proteins, meaning that you don't need to eat meat every day. In fact, your body will transform excess protein into glucose, which could make it harder to reach ketosis.

Unprocessed meats are the perfect keto choice, as they are low carb and healthy. Processed meats such as sausages and meatballs might contain added carbs. For this reason, it is recommended to make your own delicious meat-based recipes at home.

Fish and Seafood

All these are good, but fatty fish such as salmon is even better. You can enjoy your favourite fish and seafood as you want, but avoid breading, as it is usually full of carbs.

Dairy Products and Eggs

Since milk might have some hidden carbs, butter, cheese and heavy cream are perfect keto-friendly alternatives. You can still use milk sparingly in your coffee, although you should always make sure to remain within your daily intake of carbs. It goes without saying that you should avoid all dairy-based beverages, such as cappuccino, and low-fat yoghurts. This will also help you cut away lots of added sugar.

Eggs can be eaten freely. Organic or pastured eggs are usually the healthiest option. However, you should avoid eating too many eggs if you are concerned about your levels of cholesterol.

Vegetables

Fresh vegetables are healthier, but frozen food is always a decent alternative even on a keto diet.

To make the most out of your keto adventure, you must choose veggies growing above the ground, with leaves and green items. This includes cabbage, broccoli, avocado, zucchini and cauliflower.

Veggies are the best way to replace pasta, bread, rice and potatoes. This means that you could follow a vegetarian or even vegan keto diet.

Nuts and Berries

Nuts can be eaten in moderation. Cashews in particular should be avoided because they are high in carbs. You can have macadamia or pecan nuts, although you should maintain your daily intake to less than 50 grams per day.

Berries are keto-friendly, especially if accompanied by some whipping cream.

Natural Fats

When on a keto diet, the majority of your daily calories should come from fat. This can either be meat, fish, dairy or eggs. However, you should always use fat when cooking. For example, you can use butter or coconut oil, or season your salad with some extra virgin olive oil.

Some high-fat sauces, such as garlic butter and mayonnaise, can also be eaten. Although saturated fats are fine to eat on a keto diet, when it comes to industrial sauces you should always check the ingredients list to investigate potential hidden carbs.

What to Drink on A Ketogenic Diet?

Water

Water will be a powerful ally when you first approach the keto diet. Drinking plenty of water will help you feel better and avoid many of the symptoms of the keto flu. More importantly, keeping yourself hydrated is essential to help your body reach ketosis.

Coffee and Tea

Just like all other weight-loss diets, keto requires you to drink your coffee and tea without sugar. You can add a very small amount of milk or cream – no more than one tablespoon. If your drink is too bitter, you can add some butter or coconut oil, to any other keto-friendly sweeteners available on the market.

Broth

Broth is delicious, hydrating, full of nutrients, and will help you feel full. Homemade broth can be the perfect hot beverage to sip to avoid sugar cravings. Stir in a bit of butter for extra texture.

What to Avoid on A Ketogenic Diet?

Food

As a general rule, you need to avoid all low-fat diet products. Your diet should be a combination of foods which are moderately high in protein and high in fat and, of course, low in carbs.

Drink

Milk should be avoided, although you can add a small splash to your coffee or tea. Be always aware of the carbs that might hide in industrial beverages, such as readymade coffees and lattes.

When it comes to alcohol, vodka and whiskey contain zero carbs, but you should watch out for mixed drinks because they may contain huge amounts of sugar. Wine is usually lower in carbs than beer but you shouldn't drink it every day.

Can I Still Eat Bread on A Keto Diet?

One of the pillars of the keto diet is cutting down your daily intake of carbs. This will help your body get into ketosis after a few days, which will lead to weight loss and other health benefits. As you might already know, bread, pasta and rice are some of the best sources of carbs. In other words, you must avoid these foods to follow the keto diet.

On the other hand, this doesn't mean that you must say goodbye to good food! You can still enjoy your meals and eat plenty of delicious and genuine recipes that you can easily make at home. If you still like the idea of eating bread, or if you are hosting dinner and you want to serve keto-friendly bread to your guests, you can try the following recipe.

KETO-FRIENDLY BREAD

DIFFICULTY: EASY ¦ CALORIES: 165 ¦ SERVES: 6 BUNS

CARBS: 2 G ¦ FAT: 12 G ¦ PROTEIN: 6 G

INGREDIENTS

- 50 g ground psyllium husk powder
- 240 ml water
- 140 g almond flour
- 3 egg whites
- 2 tsp baking powder
- 2 tsp cider vinegar
- 1 tsp salt
- 2 tbsp sesame seeds (optional)

PREPARATION

1. Preheat the oven to 175 C and grease a baking tray.
2. Bring the water to the boil in a saucepan.
3. Meanwhile, mix all the dry ingredients in a large bowl. Add in the egg whites and the vinegar. Combine well.
4. Pour in the boiling water, and beat the mixture with a hand mixer for ½ minute. Make sure you don't overmix the dough.
5. With wet hands (you can use water or olive oil), shape the dough into 6 rolls. Transfer to the baking tray. Top with sesame seeds (optional).
6. Bake for 1 hour and enjoy your low-carb, keto-friendly bread!

Can You Go Vegetarian or Vegan on A Keto Diet?

Vegetarians eat plenty of vegetables, but they avoid meat, eggs and, in the case of vegans, dairy products.

On a traditional keto diet, the majority of your daily intake of calories come from fats, which can be found in natural oils, meat and fish, and full-fat dairies. However, you can adapt your keto regimen to meet your vegetarian needs, creating a bespoke diet. You can still get ketosis and lose weight by finding new, veggie-friendly, fat sources, such as nuts, avocados, eggs, seeds, and coconut oil.

Ketosis and The Keto Diet: An Explanation

The ultimate aim of the keto diet is to reach ketosis. This helps your body burn fat and makes you feel less hungry. In some individuals, ketosis can also help keep muscles despite weight loss.

With the keto diet rising in popularity, we often hear about ketosis and its benefits. However, this process just doesn't automatically happen as soon as you reduce your daily intake of carbs. As this is a long process which is supposed to change the way our body works, it is essential to understand all its features, including how to achieve it and how to maintain it.

What Is Ketosis?

Ketosis is a process that happens when your body doesn't have adequate amounts of carbohydrates to burn for energy. This means that it will start burning fat. This process generates ketones, which are used for fuelling your body.

When Does Ketosis Happen?

If you follow the ketogenic alimentary regimen correctly, ketosis should kick after 3 or 4 days. To reach this status, you must eat fewer than 50 grams of carbs per day. The same result can be achieved by fasting, although this isn't recommended for the majority of individuals.

Ketosis Health Benefits

Studies have demonstrated that ketosis might have some benefits and it is not only a good process to lose weight. For example, ketosis can help prevent seizures in children with epilepsy.

Research also suggests that ketosis might help people who suffer from the following diseases:

- Heart diseases
- Insulin resistance
- Metabolic syndrome
- Type 2 diabetes
- Acne
- Certain types of cancer
- Nervous system diseases, such as Parkinson's and Alzheimer's diseases
- PCOS (Polycystic ovary syndrome)

Ketosis Side Effects: The "Keto Flu"

Although ketosis can be beneficial for our body, it isn't uncommon to suffer from several side effects, especially during the first week. Don't forget that ketosis is a long process which aims to change the way your body works and processes food and energy.

This means that your body might need some time to get used to ketosis. This is what is commonly known as "keto flu". Despite its name, this isn't an official medical condition, and you shouldn't need the help of a medical professional to feel better.

Doctors believe that the period of discomfort following the first day of ketosis is linked to sugar and carbs withdrawal. It can also be due to the reaction of your immune system and gut bacteria to your new lifestyle. You should drink plenty of water during your keto flu, and you will soon feel better.

Keto flu's symptoms are temporary and should disappear within a few days. They include:
- Headache
- Brain fog and fatigue
- Irritability
- Trouble sleeping
- Constipation
- Dizziness and stomach ache

- ❧ Sore muscles and cramps
- ❧ Sugar cravings
- ❧ Bad breath (more commonly known as ketosis breath)

How to Check Your Ketosis?

To check whether your body has reached ketosis or your levels of ketones by testing your blood or urine. Of course, testing your urine is quicker and easier, and doesn't require seeking the help of a medical professional.

You can buy test strips to check your urine at home from many shops or online. You might also be able to test your levels of ketosis with some blood sugar meters.

If you find out that your levels of ketones are too high, you should talk with your doctor, as you might be at risk of ketoacidosis.

Ketosis vs. Ketoacidosis

If you follow a standard balanced diet, your body doesn't produce any ketones. However, once you cut way back on your intake of calories or carbs, your body will be forced to switch to ketosis to get more energy.

Ketosis is usually a safe process and can lead to weight loss. However, if you have diabetes and you control your ketosis, ketones will start building up and this may become dangerous. High levels of ketosis lead to dehydration and can change the chemical balance of your blood. As a result, your blood will become more acidic, and this can cause a coma or even death.

People who suffer from diabetes and don't follow a proper diet can get ketoacidosis, also known as diabetic ketoacidosis (DKA). This happens when you don't take enough insulin, or enough liquids to keep you hydrated. On the other hand, ketoacidosis might also occur if you drink too much alcohol, don't eat enough calories or suffer from certain diseases.

As a general rule, ketosis doesn't lead to ketoacidosis. However, if you have diabetes or if you are concerned about your health, you should call your doctor.

What Are the Benefits of The Keto Diet?

The keto diet works by helping your body break down fat for energy, using all its sugar reserves. The result of this process is known as ketosis, and it leads to weight loss.

However, there are several other benefits your body can enjoy by switching to a keto-friendly lifestyle. Let's find out more.

Weight Loss

It has been confirmed that the ketogenic diet can promote weight loss by boosting your metabolism and reducing the overall appetite. In other words, the food you are going to eat will fill your app easily, and reduce all those annoying hunger-stimulating hormones.

Several studies have demonstrated that people following a ketogenic diet lost weight quicker than those who weren't.

Improved Heart Health

Those who follow a ketogenic diet are more likely to eat healthful foods, which can improve your heart health and reduce cholesterol.

Studies have confirmed that those who regularly follow a ketogenic regimen have experienced significant drops in their levels of total cholesterol, bad cholesterol, and triglycerides. This translates into lower risks of heart complications.

Reduced Risk of Certain Cancers

Several pieces of research have focused on the effects of the keto diet in helping prevent or treat certain types of cancer.

One study, in particular, has found that this alimentary regimen could be useful for patients who are treating their cancer with chemotherapy and radiation therapy. The reason, as highlighted by a study from 2018, might be because this diet reduces blood sugar, lowering the risk of insulin complications.

Improved PCOS Symptoms

Several women suffer from Polycystic ovary syndrome (PCOS), which is a hormonal disorder that can lead to ovulatory dysfunction and other issues.

Science has demonstrated that a high-carb diet can have adverse effects in individuals with PCOS. This includes weight gain and skin problems.

A study from 2015 has demonstrated that the keto diet has improved some of the symptoms of PCOS, such as hormone balance and levels of fast insulin, in 24 weeks.

Improved Skin Appearance

Science has confirmed that, in several individuals, acne is linked to diet and blood sugar. A diet rich in processed and refined carbohydrates might alter the balance of gut bacteria, causing blood sugar levels to rise and fall significantly. This can have a devastating effect on your skin health.

According to a recent study, the ketogenic alimentary regimen could help reduce acne symptoms in several individuals.

Improved Brain Functions

A 2019 study suggested that the ketones generated by our body when following this lifestyle can provide some neuroprotective benefits. This means that the keto diet can be effective in strengthening and protecting our brain and nerve cells.

For some individuals, this translates into a lower risk of better management conditions for many conditions, including Alzheimer's disease.

Is the Keto Diet Right for Me?

If you are looking to start this diet and you are concerned about your health, you should seek advice from your doctor. It is also essential to first check if you suffer from diabetes, heart disease or hypoglycaemia.

Although at the moment there aren't many studies on the long-term benefits of this diet, research on the benefits of ketosis is evolving and improving day after day. If you don't suffer from any health conditions, the keto diet should be a safe eating pattern for you.

Who Should Not Try the Keto Diet?

Although the ketogenic diet can have several benefits for our bodies, certain individuals shouldn't significantly reduce their daily intake of calories and carbs. This includes the following categories:

- Those who take medication for diabetes, such as insulin
- Women who breastfeed
- Those who take medication for diabetes

If you fall within one of these categories but you are still interested to explore your options to try the keto diet or to switch to a healthier lifestyle, you should talk to your doctor.

Keto Main Meals

CAULIFLOWER STEAKS WITH ROASTED RED PEPPER AND OLIVE SALSA

DIFFICULTY: EASY ¦ CALORIES: 277 ¦ SERVES: 2

CARBS: 11 G ¦ FAT: 21 G ¦ PROTEIN: 9 G

INGREDIENTS

- 1 big cauliflower
- 4 black olives, pitted
- 1 roasted red pepper
- 2 tbsp olive oil
- 1 tsp capers
- 2 tbsp toasted flaked almonds
- ½ tbsp red wine vinegar
- ½ tsp smoked paprika
- 1 small handful parsley

PREPARATION

1. Preheat the oven to 200 C and prepare a baking tray.
2. Slice the cauliflower into two steaks, and save some florets for later.
3. Rub the paprika and ½ tbsp oil over the steaks and season with salt. Place onto the trash and roast for 20 minutes.
4. To make the salsa, chop the parsley, olives, peppers, and capers. Mix in a bowl and season to taste.
5. Serve the cauliflower steaks topped with salsa and flaked almonds.

STEAK WITH PORCINI BUTTER AND CHARRED ONION

DIFFICULTY: EASY ¦ CALORIES: 279 ¦ SERVES: 4

CARBS: 19 G ¦ FAT: 13 G ¦ PROTEIN: 23 G

INGREDIENTS

- 4 x 150 g minute steaks
- 100 g unsalted butter, softened
- 2 tbsp dried porcini mushrooms, chopped
- 1 bunch salad onions
- 2 garlic cloves, crushed
- 2 lemons, halved
- 2 tbsp thyme leaves
- 1 tbsp extra virgin olive oil

PREPARATION

1. Immerse the porcini in a bowl with boiling water. Once the liquid is absorbed, add garlic, thyme and butter. Season with salt and spread half of this butter over the steaks.
2. Cook the steaks for 1-2 minutes on each side until medium-rare, or cook to your liking.
3. Cover the steaks with foil and leave to rest.
4. Meanwhile, brush the onions and the lemons with olive oil and fry for 2 minutes in a hot pan.
5. Serve the steaks with lemon and onion, and the remaining mushrooms butter.

KETO JAPANESE KINGFISH LETTUCE CUPS

DIFFICULTY: EASY ¦ CALORIES: 275 ¦ SERVES: 4

CARBS: 15 G ¦ FAT: 21 G ¦ PROTEIN: 32 G

INGREDIENTS

- 800 g kingfish fillet, skin off, cut into pieces
- 2 little gem lettuces, leaves separated, shredded
- ¼ red cabbage, shredded
- 4 watermelon radishes, sliced
- 6 spring onions, sliced
- 2 tbsp light soy sauce
- 2 tbsp oyster sauce
- 2 tbsp peanut oil
- 1 garlic clove, crushed
- 1 tbsp fish sauce
- Your choice of sauce, to serve

PREPARATION

1. Place the kingfish fillet in a food processor and pulse until it is finely chopped.
2. In a frying pan, high the oil and fry the onion and garlic. After 2 minutes, add the fish and cook until starting to colour.
3. Add the soy sauce, fish sauce and oyster sauce. Leave to cook until the sauces have reduced.
4. Serve this mixture in lettuce leaves. Top with radish slices, cabbage and your choice of sauce.

CHICKEN SALAD STUFFED AVOCADO

DIFFICULTY: EASY ¦ CALORIES: 431 ¦ SERVES: 4

CARBS: 11 G ¦ FAT: 30 G ¦ PROTEIN: 31 G

INGREDIENTS

- 2 avocados, pitted
- 2 tbsp Greek yoghurt
- The juice of 1 lemon
- 150 g shredded cooked chicken
- 30 g mayonnaise
- 1 ½ tsp Dijon mustard
- ½ red onion, minced
- Chopped parsley, to garnish

PREPARATION

1. Scoop out avocados, but make sure to leave a small border. Dice the avocado flesh.
2. To make the chicken salad, mix the meat, onion, yoghurt, mayo, mustard and lemon juice in a bowl. Add in the diced avocado and season with salt and pepper to taste.
3. Serve the salad into the 4 avocado halves, and garnish with chopped parsley.

KETO CAULIFLOWER CHOWDER

DIFFICULTY: EASY ¦ CALORIES: 288 ¦ SERVES: 6-8

CARBS: 12 G ¦ FAT: 16 G ¦ PROTEIN: 15 G

INGREDIENTS

- 4 slices bacon, cut into pieces
- 2 medium carrots, peeled and chopped
- 1 l vegetable broth
- 1 medium yellow onion, chopped
- 1 head cauliflower, cut into florets
- 2 stalk celery, chopped
- 2 cloves garlic, minced
- 2 tbsp flour
- 2 sprigs thyme, chopped
- 60 ml whole milk

PREPARATION

1. Cook the bacon in a large pot until crispy. Transfer to a plate lined with a paper towel and drain part of the excess fat.
2. In the same pot, cook the celery, carrots and onion. Season to taste. Add in the garlic and the flour and stir well for 2 minutes. Add cauliflower and thyme.
3. Pour in the milk and vegetable broth and bring to a boil. Reduce heat and leave to simmer for 15 minutes.
4. Garnish with bacon and season to taste.

LOW-CARB PUMPKIN SPAGHETTI

DIFFICULTY: EASY ¦ CALORIES: 144 ¦ SERVES: 4

CARBS: 4 G ¦ FAT: 12 G ¦ PROTEIN: 22 G

INGREDIENTS

- 1 butternut pumpkin, halved, seeds removed
- 2 garlic cloves, sliced
- 1 bunch sage, leaves picked
- 4 sliced ham, torn into pieces
- 60 g butter, chopped
- 55 g almonds, chopped
- Extra almonds, to serve
- Your choice of sauce

PREPARATION

1. Preheat the oven to 250 C.
2. With a mandolin or a spiraliser, turn your pumpkin into spaghetti.
3. Spread the sage leaves, ham, almonds and garlic onto a roasting pan. Scatter butter.
4. Add in the pumpkin spaghetti and bake for 10-15 minutes.
5. Top with extra almonds and serve with your choice of keto-friendly sauce.

KETO CHILI

DIFFICULTY: MEDIUM ¦ CALORIES: 435 ¦ SERVES: 8

CARBS: 11G ¦ FAT: 33 G ¦ PROTEIN: 25 G

INGREDIENTS

- 1 kg ground beef
- 3 slices bacon, cut into strips
- 1 green bell pepper, chopped
- 2 celery stalks, chopped
- ¼ medium yellow onion, chopped
- 2 cloves garlic, minced
- 2 tbsp smoked paprika
- 2 tsp dried oregano
- 2 tbsp chilli powder
- 2 tsp ground cumin
- 300 ml beef broth
- 60 g mushrooms, sliced
- Shredded cheddar, to garnish
- Sour cream, to garnish
- Sliced avocado, to garnish
- Sliced green onions, to garnish

PREPARATION

1. Cook the bacon in a pot over medium heat. Remove from heat once crispy.
2. In the same pot, cook the pepper, celery, onion, and mushrooms. Add the garlic and cook until fragrant.
3. Add the beef and cook well.
4. Stir in the cumin, oregano, chilli powder and paprika. Season to taste.
5. Add the broth and bring to a simmer, then cook for 15 minutes.
6. Serve into bowls, topped with sour cream, cheese, avocado and green onions.

SPINACH & RICOTTA GNOCCHI

DIFFICULTY: MEDIUM ¦ CALORIES: 287 ¦ SERVES: 4

CARBS: 19 G ¦ FAT: 15 G ¦ PROTEIN: 20 G

INGREDIENTS

- 200 g spinach, washed
- 2 eggs
- 85 g plain flour
- 140 g ricotta
- 1 garlic clove, crushed
- 1 small handful parsley leaves, chopped
- 100 g parmesan (or any vegetarian alternative)
- Freshly grated nutmeg
- Olive oil, to serve
- Rocket, to serve

PREPARATION

1. Place the spinach in a bowl in boiling water. Leave for 2 minutes, then drain and allow to cool. Remove extra liquid with a clean tea towel.
2. In a large bowl, mix the spinach, eggs, ricotta, parsley, garlic, cheese and nutmeg. Season with salt and pepper. With a fork, stir thoroughly until everything is perfectly mixed. With wed hands, form the egg mixture into balls. Refrigerate for at least ½ hour.
3. Once ready to cook, bring a pan of water to the boil.
4. Cook the gnocchi for about 1-2 minutes.
5. Serve the gnocchi drizzled with olive oil, rocket and extra cheese.

KETO-FRIENDLY CRUSTLESS QUICHE

DIFFICULTY: MEDIUM ¦ CALORIES: 401 ¦ SERVES: 6

CARBS: 3 G ¦ FAT: 34 G ¦ PROTEIN: 19 G

INGREDIENTS

- 100 g chopped pancetta (or smoked bacon)
- 200 g asparagus, trimmed (or broccoli)
- 20 g butter
- 150 g double cream
- 80 g parmesan cheese (or gruyere)
- 8 large eggs
- 1 onion, chopped

PREPARATION

1. Heat oven to 180 C and prepare a cake tin.
2. Melt the butter in a pan. Add in the pancetta and onion and cook for 10 minutes.
3. Bring a pan of salted water to the boil to cook the asparagus (or the broccoli).
4. In a bowl, whisk the cream, eggs and 2/3 of the cheese. Season with salt and pepper. Add in the onion and bacon.
5. Pour the mixture into the tip. Top with the vegetables and sprinkle the remaining cheese. Bake for ½ hour.

KETO WEST INDIAN SPICED AUBERGINE CURRY

DIFFICULTY: MEDIUM ¦ CALORIES: 157 ¦ SERVES: 2

CARBS: 13 G ¦ FAT: 9 G ¦ PROTEIN: 4 G

INGREDIENTS

- 1 large aubergine
- 2 tbsp tomato puree
- 3 spring onions, chopped
- 1 tsp ground coriander
- 1 tsp ground cumin
- 1 cm piece of ginger, peeled and chopped
- 1 ½ tbsp rapeseed oil
- 2 tsp caster sugar
- ½ tsp ground turmeric
- ½ bunch coriander, shredded
- ½ green chilli, chopped
- Cooked cauliflower rice, to serve
- Natural full-fat yoghurt, to serve
- Lime wedges, to serve

PREPARATION

1. Mix all the dry spices with 1 tsp salt in a bowl.
2. Slice the aubergine and score both sides with the tip of a knife. Rub with the spice mix.
3. In a bowl, put 150 ml water, chilli, tomato puree, sugar and ginger.
4. Heat the oil in a pan and cook the aubergine for 5 minutes on each side. Add the tomato puree mix and cook for 15-20 minutes. Add more water if necessary. Season to taste.
5. Serve the aubergine scattered over with spring onions and coriander. Serve with cauliflower rice, yoghurt and lime wedges.

LOW-CARB CAULIFLOWER PIZZA

DIFFICULTY: MEDIUM ¦ CALORIES: 354 ¦ SERVES: 1 PIZZA

CARBS: 18 G ¦ FAT: 15 G ¦ PROTEIN: 13 G

INGREDIENTS

- 60 ml tomato pasta sauce
- 100 g mozzarella, thinly sliced
- 60 ml pesto

Cauliflower dough

- 1 big cauliflower
- 30 g grated parmesan
- 75 g almonds
- 2 eggs
- 1 tbsp olive oil

- 250 mixed cherry tomatoes, halved
- Baby basil leaves, to garnish

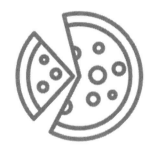

PREPARATION

1. Preheat the oven to 140 C and prepare two baking trays with baking paper.

2. Chop the cauliflower and use a food processor to pulse until it is finely chopped. Using a clean cloth, squeeze and remove all the excess liquid and moisture.

3. Spread the cauliflower over the trays and bake for 15 minutes. Once completely dried out, leave to cool.

4. Return the cauliflower to the food processor and add the almonds, parmesan, and the eggs. Season with salt and pepper. Process until you get a smooth dough.

5. Spread the cauliflower mixture to the baking tray. Increase oven to 180 C and roast for 25/30 minutes, or until golden.

6. Increase the oven once again to 250 C. Spread the pesto and tomato sauce over the cauliflower base and top with mozzarella. Roast for additional 10 minutes, or until the cheese is melted.

7. Garnish with basil leaves and serve your delicious pizza.

KETO GINGER CHICKEN STIR-FRY

DIFFICULTY: MEDIUM ¦ CALORIES: 411 ¦ SERVES: 4

CARBS: 15 G ¦ FAT: 39 G ¦ PROTEIN: 24 G

INGREDIENTS

- 700 g boneless chicken thighs, cut into pieces
- 300 g broccoli, cut into florets
- 4 spring onions, cut into batons
- 5 shiitake mushrooms, sliced
- 2 baby bok choy, chopped
- 1 carrot, cut into matchsticks
- 3 tbsp coconut oil

Stir-Fry Sauce

- 6 cm piece of ginger, cut into matchsticks
- 4 garlic cloves, chopped
- 1 tbsp coconut oil
- 250 ml chicken broth
- 1 long red chilli, cut into matchsticks
- 2 tbsp toasted sesame oil
- 1 tbsp coconut sugar
- 3 tbsp tamari
- 2 tsp sesame seeds
- 2 tsp tapioca flour

Cauliflower Rice

- 1 head cauliflower
- 2 tbsp coconut oil
- Salt and pepper

PREPARATION

1. To make the stir-fry sauce, heat the coconut oil over medium heat. Add in the garlic, chilli and ginger. Cook for 1 minute. Pour in the tamari and chicken broth, coconut sugar, pepper, and sesame seeds. Bring to a simmer. Add in the tapioca mixture and bring to the boil. Once ready, set aside.

2. Melt 1 tbsp coconut oil in a wok and stir fry the chicken for 5 minutes. Transfer to a plate.

3. Stir fry the spring onion in the remaining coconut oil. Add the other vegetables and cook for 5 minutes.

4. Return the chicken to the pan, pour in the stir fry sauce, and cook everything together for 2 minutes. Season with salt and pepper, if needed.

5. To make the cauliflower rice, place the florets in a food processor and pulse until you get a fine rice-like texture. Heat the coconut oil and stir fry the cauliflower rice for a few minutes. Season with salt and pepper.

6. Serve the cauliflower rice topped with the stir fry mixture, extra sesame seeds and coriander leaves.

Healthy and Indulgent Keto Salads

KETO COBB EGG SALAD

DIFFICULTY: EASY ¦ CALORIES: 217 ¦ SERVES: 6

CARBS: 8 G ¦ FAT: 16 G ¦ PROTEIN: 29 G

INGREDIENTS

- 8 hard-boiled eggs, cut into eight pieces
- 1 avocado, sliced
- 8 strips bacon, crumbled
- 2 tbsp red wine vinegar
- 3 tbsp Greek full-fat yoghurt
- 3 tbsp mayonnaise
- 2 tbsp freshly chopped chives
- 50 g blue cheese, crumbled (plus extra to garnish)
- 8-10 cherry tomatoes, halved

PREPARATION

1. Mix the mayonnaise, red wine vinegar and yoghurt in a bowl. Season with salt and pepper.
2. In another bowl, mix the eggs, avocado, bacon, blue cheese and tomatoes.
3. Gently fold the mayonnaise dressing into the eggs bowl.
4. Garnish with chives, extra cheese, and your choice of toppings, or extra tomatoes.

KETO RED-BRAISED PORK BELLY WITH APPLE SALAD

DIFFICULTY: EASY ¦ CALORIES: 234 ¦ SERVES: 4

CARBS: 21 G ¦ FAT: 19 G ¦ PROTEIN: 27 G

INGREDIENTS

- 1.2 kg boneless pork belly, cut into pieces
- 250 ml light soy sauce
- 500 ml dark soy sauce
- 10 cm piece of ginger, sliced
- 1 bunch spring onions
- 10 star anise
- 1 kg caster sugar
- 3 cinnamon quills
- 2 Granny Smith apples, cut into matchsticks
- The juice of 1 lemon
- 1 bunch coriander, leaves picked
- 2 tbsp olive oil

PREPARATION

1. Place the pork belly, skin-side up, in a dish and sprinkle with salt. Refrigerate for 2 hours.

2. Mix the sugar, ginger, spices, green spring onions, and soy sauces in a stockpot. Cover with water and leave to simmer until the sugar dissolves. Cover with a lid and leave to simmer for at least 1 hour.

3. Add the pork to the stockpot. Reduce the heat and leave to simmer for 2 hours.

4. Leave the pork to cool, then cut into cubes.

5. To make the salad, combine extra spring onions with the apple and coriander. Season with salt, lemon juice and oil.

6. Serve the pork belly with the apple salad and a spoonful of stock.

KETO AUTUMN VEGETABLE SALAD WITH SAFFRON DRESSING

DIFFICULTY: EASY ¦ CALORIES: 167 ¦ SERVES: 6

CARBS: 9 G ¦ FAT: 12 G ¦ PROTEIN: 3 G

INGREDIENTS

- 12 rainbow carrots, peeled
- 8 stalks long-stem broccoli, halved lengthways
- ½ cucumber cut lengthwise
- 1 medium courgette, sliced
- 4 spring onions, sliced
- 100 g mixed cherry tomatoes, halved
- 3 plum tomatoes, peeled and cut into pieces
- 1 tbsp rapeseed oil
- 30 g black olives, stoned and sliced
- 3 tbsp basil, roughly chopped

Dressing

- 50 ml extra virgin rapeseed oil
- 20 ml cider vinegar
- 1 tsp caster sugar
- ½ tsp Dijon mustard
- 1 small shallot, chopped
- 1 pinch of saffron strands

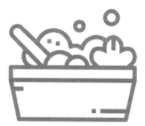

PREPARATION

1. Heat a pan over medium heat. Stir in the courgette, carrots and broccoli in rapeseed oil. Stir-fry for 3 minutes, then transfer to a bowl.
2. Add the remaining salad ingredients in a bowl and toss together.
3. To make the dressing, whisk the sugar, saffron, vinegar and mustard together. Season with a pinch of salt and keep whisking until the sugar dissolves. Add in the oil gradually, then the shallots.
4. Serve the salad tossed with the dressing.

TOMATO, BURRATA AND BEAN SALAD

DIFFICULTY: EASY ¦ CALORIES: 409 ¦ SERVES: 4

CARBS: 7 G ¦ FAT: 32 G ¦ PROTEIN: 22 G

INGREDIENTS

- 500 g tomatoes
- 2 x 100 g burrata
- 150 g broad beans, podded
- 50 g hazelnuts, toasted and chopped
- ½ tsp caster sugar
- 1 tbsp lovage
- 1 tbsp tarragon
- 1 tbsp red wine vinegar
- 2 tsp Dijon mustard
- 3 tbsp olive oil
- 1 tbsp mint leaves
- The zest of 1 lemon
- 1 pinch of fennel seeds
- Handful flat-leaf parsley
- Handful basil

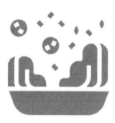

PREPARATION

1. Cut the tomatoes into wedges, and transfer to a bowl. Toss with a pinch of salt and the sugar. Leave to marinate for ½ hour.

2. Meanwhile, bring a pan of water to the boil and cook the beans for 2 minutes. Drain well and allow to cool.

3. Peel the beans out of their shells.

4. Chop the herbs and add into the bowl with the tomatoes. With the mustard, lemon zest, fennel seeds, olive oil and the red wine vinegar. Season with salt if necessary and add in the beans.

5. Transfer to a serving plate. Top with the burrata and the beans. Scatter over the hazelnuts and extra lemon zest if you want.

ASPARAGUS SALAD WITH POACHED EGG

DIFFICULTY: EASY ¦ CALORIES: 228 ¦ SERVES: 2

CARBS: 13 G ¦ FAT: 13 G ¦ PROTEIN: 13 G

INGREDIENTS

- 8 asparagus spears, trimmed
- 2 large eggs
- 200 g cooked beetroot, peeled and cut into pieces
- ¼ cucumber, cut into batons
- 1 tbsp balsamic vinegar
- 1 tbsp extra virgin olive oil
- 2 handfuls mixed leaves

PREPARATION

1. Pour the vinegar and olive oil into a small bowl. Add in the beetroot and mix well.
2. Divide the cucumber and mixed leaves into 2 serving plates.
3. Cook the asparagus in simmering water for a couple of minutes.
4. Crack the eggs into a hot pan and cook for a few minutes, until the yolks are just beginning to set.
5. Add the eggs to the salad, pour over the dressing and top with asparagus and a poached egg.

KETO SHRIMPO DE GALLO

DIFFICULTY: EASY ¦ CALORIES: 275 ¦ SERVES: 8

CARBS: 16 G ¦ FAT: 23 G ¦ PROTEIN: 24 G

INGREDIENTS

- 500 g large shrimps, tails removed
- 1 clove garlic, minced
- 1 avocado, diced
- ½ white onion, chopped
- 30 g chopped cilantro
- 500 g tomatoes, diced
- 1 tbsp extra virgin olive oil
- 2 tbsp fresh lime juice
- ¼ tsp chilli powder
- 2 jalapeno peppers, seeds removed, diced

PREPARATION

1. Heat the oil in a large skillet over medium heat. Cook the shrimps and season with garlic and chilli powder. Transfer to a cutting board.
2. Roughly chop the shrimps into small pieces and transfer into a bowl. Add in the onion, tomatoes, cilantro, lime juice, jalapeno and avocado. Season with salt and pepper to taste.
3. Mix well and serve.

PARMESAN AND BRUSSEL SPROUTS SALAD

DIFFICULTY: EASY ¦ CALORIES: 269 ¦ SERVES: 6

CARBS: 12 G ¦ FAT: 19 G ¦ PROTEIN: 16 G

INGREDIENTS

- 900 g Brussel sprouts, halved and sliced
- 130 g freshly chopped parsley
- 5 tbsp lemon juice
- 5 tbsp extra virgin olive oil
- 60 g pomegranate seeds
- 60 g chopped toasted almonds
- Shaved parmesan, to serve

PREPARATION

1. Whisk the oil, lemon juice, parsley, salt and pepper in a bowl.
2. Add in the Brussel sprouts and toss until well coated. Let sit for at least 20 minutes.
3. Add in the pomegranate seeds and almonds.
4. Serve with shaved parmesan.

KETO STRAWBERRY AND SPINACH SALAD

DIFFICULTY: EASY ¦ CALORIES: 199 ¦ SERVES: 4

CARBS: 12 G ¦ FAT: 23 G ¦ PROTEIN: 18 G

INGREDIENTS

- 250 g baby spinach
- ¼ red onion, sliced
- 50 g feta, crumbled
- 10 g chopped toasted pecans
- 2 chicken breasts, cooked and cut into pieces
- 2 tbsp fresh lemon juice
- 1 tbsp extra virgin olive oil
- ½ tsp Dijon mustard
- 120 g strawberries, thinly sliced

PREPARATION

1. Whisk the lemon juice and the mustard in a bowl. Pour in the oil and mix the dressing until well combined.
2. Add in the chicken, spinach, strawberries, ½ of the pecans, and onion. Toss to combine with the dressing.
3. Transfer to serving plates and serve with the remaining pecans and crumbling feta.

KETO CAPRESE SALAD

DIFFICULTY: EASY ¦ CALORIES: 174 ¦ SERVES: 4-6

CARBS: 7 G ¦ FAT: 13 G ¦ PROTEIN: 21 G

INGREDIENTS

- 450 g fresh mozzarella
- 6 medium ripe tomatoes, sliced
- 1 bunch fresh basil, stems removed
- 1 tbsp extra virgin olive oil

PREPARATION

1. Layer the mozzarella and tomato slices on a large serving plate.
2. Drizzle with olive oil.
3. Season with salt and pepper.

KETO CRISPY PORK BELLY SALAD WITH MINT AND CORIANDER

DIFFICULTY: EASY ¦ CALORIES: 389 ¦ SERVES: 4

CARBS: 19 G ¦ FAT: 33 G ¦ PROTEIN: 26 G

INGREDIENTS

- 1 kg boneless pork belly, with skin, scored at 1 cm intervals all over
- 1 small cucumber, sliced
- 3 spring onions, sliced
- 1 red chilli, seeds removed, chopped
- 2 tbsp lime juice
- ¼ cup basil leaves
- ¼ cup mint leaves
- 2 tbsp chopped salted peanuts
- ¼ coriander leaves
- 2 tbsp fish sauce
- 2 tsp caster sugar

PREPARATION

1. Preheat the oven to 200 C.
2. Remove excess moisture from the pork skin with a paper towel, then rub all over with salt.
3. Place the pork skin-side up in a roasting pan, cover with water and roast for 2 hours, covering with additional water if necessary. Once ready, set the pork aside and allow to cool, then cut the meat into bite-sized pieces.
4. In a bowl, mix the lime juice, sugar and fish sauce, until the sugar dissolves. Add in the pork, cucumber, spring onion, chilli and herbs. Toss to combine well.
5. Serve the salad with scattered peanuts.

SEARED TUNA AND CUCUMBER SALAD

DIFFICULTY: MEDIUM ¦ CALORIES: 254 ¦ SERVES: 6-8

CARBS: 9 G ¦ FAT: 11 G ¦ PROTEIN: 29 G

INGREDIENTS

- 400 g yellowfin tuna steaks
- 2 tbsp sesame oil
- 1 tbsp sunflower oil

- 3 tbsp soy sauce
- 1 tbsp cracked black pepper

Salad

- 3 cucumber, peeled, halved, and spiralised
- 8 breakfast radishes, trimmed and sliced
- 1 mooli, peeled and spiralised (or use 2 extra breakfast radishes)
- 1 small piece ginger, peeled and cut into matchsticks

- 2 sheets nori, cut into strips
- 3 tbsp mirin
- 1 red chilli, deseeded and chopped
- 1 tbsp coriander seeds, toasted and crushed
- 1 large bunch coriander, chopped
- 2 tbsp sushi ginger, chopped (optional)

Dressing

- 1 tsp soy sauce
- 4 tbsp natural full-fat yoghurt
- The juice of 1 lime
- 1 tsp wasabi

PREPARATION

1. Whisk the sesame oil, soy sauce and pepper together.
2. Heat the sunflower oil in a frying pan and sear the tuna steaks on both sides until well cooked. Transfer to the sesame oil mixture and leave to marinate for 1 h. Turn the steaks and continue to chill.
3. Meanwhile, to make the salad, mix all the vegetables into a large bowl. Add the ginger and the nori. Drizzle over the lime juice and mirin, then add in the chilli and coriander.
4. To make the dressing, whisk all ingredients together.
5. Serve the tuna with the salad drizzled over with the dressing, and sprinkle over the coriander seeds.

BARBECUED BAVETTE STEAK AND TOMATO SALAD

DIFFICULTY: MEDIUM ¦ CALORIES: 253 ¦ SERVES: 6-8

CARBS: 6 G ¦ FAT: 16 G ¦ PROTEIN: 19 G

INGREDIENTS

- 500 g mixed heritage tomatoes
- 200 g grilled artichokes in oil, drained
- 500 g bavette steak

Dressing

- 3 spring onions, sliced
- 2 tbsp red wine vinegar
- 3 tbsp olive oil
- 1 tsp onion seeds

- 150 g feta, crumbled
- 2 tbsp olive oil
- 2 red onions, cut into slices
- ½ bunch chives, shipped

PREPARATION

1. To make the dressing, whisk the onion seeds, vinegar, spring onions in a bowl.
2. Slice the tomatoes and transfer to a serving platter. Season with salt and drizzle with some oil.
3. Heat a pan and cook the steak for 2-3 minutes on each side. Leave to rest on a plate.
4. Drizzle the remaining oil over the onions, separated into rings, and grill for a few minutes.
5. Slice the steak and serve with the tomatoes over it. Drizzle with the resting juice and top with onions, artichokes, feta and chives. Serve with the dressing.

KETO CHICKEN SOUVLAKI WITH GREEK SALAD

DIFFICULTY: CHALLENGING ¦ CALORIES: 279 ¦ SERVES: 4

CARBS: 15 G ¦ FAT: 16 G ¦ PROTEIN: 17 G

INGREDIENTS

- 8 boneless chicken thighs, skin on, cut into cubes
- Salt and pepper
- Lemon wedges, to serve

Keto Tzatziki

- 200 g coconut yoghurt
- ½ cucumber, grated
- 1 tbsp mint leaves, finely chopped
- 1 tbsp extra virgin olive oil
- 1 garlic clove, finely grated
- 1 tsp dill fronds, finely chopped
- 1 tsp lemon juice

Marinade

- The juice of 2 lemon
- 3 tbsp coconut oil, melted
- 1 tbsp red wine vinegar
- ½ tsp sweet paprika
- 1 tbsp garlic, finely grated
- 1 tsp ground cumin
- 1 tsp dried thyme
- 2 ½ tsp dried oregano
- 1 tsp honey (optional)

Greek Salad

- 1 cucumber, halved and sliced
- ¼ red onion, sliced
- 2 tomatoes, cut into wedges
- 1 baby lettuce, quartered
- 3 tbsp extra virgin olive oil
- 2 tbsp red wine vinegar

Coconut Yogurt

- 1.2 l coconut cream
- 1 tbsp powdered gelatine
- 2 tbsp filtered water
- 4 probiotic capsules
- 1 tbsp lemon juice (optional)
- 2 tbsp honey or coconut sugar (optional)

PREPARATION

1. Start with the coconut yoghurt. Wash and prepare a 1.5 l preserving jar with a lid. Place the water in a bowl and sprinkle over the gelatine. Leave to soak for 2 minutes. Heat the vanilla seeds and coconut cream in a saucepan. Stir often until it starts to simmer. Remove from the pan and set aside to cool. Pour 125 ml of this coconut cream into a sterilised bowl and stir in the probiotic powder from the capsules and the lemon juice. Add the remaining mixture and stir well. Pour everything into the jar, seal with the lid and leave to ferment in a warm place for at least 12 hours. Once ready, stir well and refrigerate for at least 5 hours.

2. To make the tzatziki, combine all the ingredients in a bowl and season with salt if needed. Cover and place in the fridge for a few minutes.

3. To make the marinade, combine all the ingredients. Season with salt and pepper.

4. Add the chicken cubes to the marinade and mix until well coated. Place in the fridge and leave to marinate for 2 hours.

5. Once ready, thread the marinated chicken onto some wooden or bamboo skewers. Season with salt and pepper.

6. Cook on a chargrill pan or barbecue grill plate for 15 minutes or until cooked through.

7. Make the salad by mixing all the ingredients in a bowl.

8. Serve the chicken skewers with all the other sauces and the yoghurt, plus extra lemon wedges and the Greek salad.

Perfect Keto-Friendly Soups

THAI CHICKEN COCONUT SOUP

DIFFICULTY: EASY ¦ CALORIES: 211 ¦ SERVES: 4

CARBS: 16 G ¦ FAT: 24 G ¦ PROTEIN: 11 G

INGREDIENTS

- 300 ml chicken broth
- 450 g boneless, skinless chicken thighs, cut into pieces
- 115 g shiitake mushrooms, chopped
- 1 tbsp fish sauce
- 1 can coconut milk
- 1 tbsp freshly minced ginger
- 1 tbsp extra virgin olive oil
- The juice of 1 lime
- Cilantro leaves, to garnish
- Chilli oil, to garnish (optional)

PREPARATION

1. Heat the oil in a pan over medium heat. Stir fry the ginger for 1 minute, then add in the mushrooms and cook for 5 minutes.
2. Add coconut milk, fish sauce, and broth. Bring to the boil. Add the chicken and leave to simmer for 15 minutes, or until it is no longer pink.
3. Turn the heat off. Stir in the lime juice.
4. Serve the chicken soup garnished with cilantro and chilli oil (optional).

KETO-FRIENDLY CAULIFLOWER SOUP

DIFFICULTY: EASY ¦ CALORIES: 176 ¦ SERVES: 4-6

CARBS: 14 G ¦ FAT: 38 G ¦ PROTEIN: 8 G

INGREDIENTS

- 1 large cauliflower, cut into florets
- 850 ml vegetable stock
- 100 ml single cream
- 1 garlic clove, crushed
- 1 celery stick, chopped
- 4 thyme sprigs
- 1 onion, chopped
- 2 tbsp olive oil
- ½ tbsp ground cumin
- ½ small bunch of parsley, chopped

PREPARATION

1. Heat the oven to 200 C.
2. Spread the cauliflower florets in a roasting tin and drizzle with 1 tbsp olive oil, thyme and cumin. Roast for 15 minutes. Discard the thyme once ready.
3. Heat the remaining oil in a saucepan and fry the onion and celery over medium heat for 10 minutes, or until softened. Add in the garlic and ¾ of the cauliflower. Add the stock and bring to a simmer. Cook for 10-12 minutes.
4. With a food processor, pulse the cauliflower mixture until smooth.
5. Season to taste and serve with the reserved cauliflower, parsley, and extra olive oil.

BROCCOLI CHEDDAR SOUP

DIFFICULTY: EASY ¦ CALORIES: 231 ¦ SERVES: 4

CARBS: 11 G ¦ FAT: 18 G ¦ PROTEIN: 5 G

INGREDIENTS

- 1 small onion, diced
- 2 small heads broccoli, cut into florets plus the stems cut into pieces
- 85 g cheddar, grated
- 3 tbsp all-purpose flour
- 60 ml half-and-half
- 120 ml vegetable broth
- 3 tbsp unsalted butter
- 1 pinch of nutmeg
- 2 cloves garlic, crushed
- Greek full-fat yoghurt or sour cream, to garnish

PREPARATION

1. Melt the butter in a medium pot over medium heat. Cook the onion for 5 minutes, then stir in the garlic and cook until fragrant. Add the flour and stir constantly for 3 minutes, or until it turns golden.
2. Add the half-and-half and the broth and bring to the boil. Reduce the heat and stir in the broccoli. Save a few pieces of broccoli for garnish. Leave to simmer for 15 minutes, or until broccoli is tender.
3. With an immersion blender, puree the soup in the pot.
4. Whisk in the cheddar and season to taste. Add the nutmeg.
5. Garnish with extra broccoli, Greek yoghurt or sour cream.

Delicious Keto-Friendly Breakfast Ideas

MUSHROOM HASH WITH POACHED EGGS

DIFFICULTY: EASY ¦ CALORIES: 283 ¦ SERVES: 4

CARBS: 15 G ¦ FAT: 17 G ¦ PROTEIN: 15 G

INGREDIENTS

- 500 g mushrooms, quartered
- 4 large eggs
- 500 g fresh tomatoes, chopped
- 4 tsp seed mix
- 2 large onions, halved and sliced
- 1 tsp smoked paprika
- 1 ½ tbsp rapeseed oil
- 1 tbsp fresh thyme leaves
- Extra thyme leaves, to garnish

PREPARATION

1. Heat the oil in a pan and stir fry the onions. Cover with a lid to leave the onions to cook in their own steam.
2. Add in the mushrooms and the thyme and cook for 5 minutes, or until softened.
3. Stir in the tomatoes and the smoked paprika. Cover with a lid and cook for 5 minutes.
4. Stir in the seed mix.
5. Poach the eggs in lightly simmering water.
6. Serve the eggs on top of the mushroom hash, with additional thyme.

SCRAMBLED EGGS WITH BASIL, SPINACH & TOMATOES

DIFFICULTY: EASY ¦ CALORIES: 297 ¦ SERVES: 2

CARBS: 10 G ¦ FAT: 17 G ¦ PROTEIN: 20 G

INGREDIENTS

- 4 large eggs
- 3 tomatoes, halved
- 175 g baby spinach
- 1/3 small pack basil, chopped
- 1 tbsp + 1 tsp rapeseed oil
- 4 tbsp natural yoghurt

PREPARATION

1. Heat 1 tsp oil in a pan and stir fry the tomatoes over medium heat.
2. Meanwhile, beat the eggs in a bowl with 2 tbsp water, the yoghurt, basil, and black pepper.
3. Transfer the tomatoes to your serving plates. In the same pan, cook the spinach for a few minutes.
4. Heat the remaining oil and pour in the egg mixture, making scrambled eggs.
5. Add the spinach and the scrambled eggs into your serving plates.

KETO MUSHROOM BRUNCH

DIFFICULTY: EASY ¦ CALORIES: 154 ¦ SERVES: 4

CARBS: 1 G ¦ FAT: 11 G ¦ PROTEIN: 13 G

INGREDIENTS

- 250 g mushrooms, sliced
- 160 g kale
- 4 medium egg
- 1 garlic clove, crushed
- 1 tbsp extra virgin olive oil

PREPARATION

1. Heat the oil in a pan and fry the garlic for 1-2 minutes. Add in the mushrooms and cook for a few minutes, or until soft. Stir in the kale.
2. Season with salt and pepper to taste.
3. Crack in the eggs and cook for 2-3 minutes. Cover the pan with a lid and cook for further 2-3 minutes.

KETO MUSHROOMS BAKED EGGS WITH SQUASHED TOMATOES

DIFFICULTY: EASY ¦ CALORIES: 147 ¦ SERVES: 2

CARBS: 5 G ¦ FAT: 8 G ¦ PROTEIN: 12 G

INGREDIENTS

- 2 large flat mushrooms, chopped
- 2 large eggs
- 2 tomatoes, halved
- ½ garlic clove, grated
- 2 handfuls rocket
- 1 tbsp rapeseed oil
- 1 few thyme leaves

PREPARATION

1. Heat oven to 200 C.
2. Brush the mushrooms with the oil and garlic, then place into two greased gratin dishes. Season with salt and pepper.
3. Top with chopped stalks and thyme. Cover with foil and bake for 20-25 minutes.
4. Once ready, remove the foil. Add the tomatoes and break an egg onto each mushroom.
5. Return to oven for 10 minutes.
6. Top with the rocket before serving.

KETO TOMATO BAKED EGGS

DIFFICULTY: EASY ¦ CALORIES: 204 ¦ SERVES: 4

CARBS: 7 G ¦ FAT: 16 G ¦ PROTEIN: 9 G

INGREDIENTS

- 900 g ripe vine tomatoes, cut into wedges
- 3 tbsp olive oil
- 3 garlic cloves, peeled and sliced
- 4 large eggs
- 2 tbsp chopped parsley

PREPARATION

1. Preheat the oven to 180 C.
2. Spread the tomato wedges over an ovenproof dish. Sprinkle with the garlic and drizzle with the oil. Season to taste.
3. Stir well and bake for 40 minutes.
4. Make four gaps among your tomatoes and break an egg into each space.
5. Return to oven for 10 minutes.
6. Scatter with herbs before serving.

KETO GREEN EGGS

DIFFICULTY: EASY ¦ CALORIES: 298 ¦ SERVES: 2

CARBS: 8 G ¦ FAT: 20 G ¦ PROTEIN: 18 G

INGREDIENTS

- 2 large eggs
- 200 g spinach
- 2 garlic cloves, sliced
- 2 tbsp Greek yoghurt
- 2 trimmed leeks, sliced
- ½ tsp fennel seeds
- ½ tsp coriander seeds
- 1 ½ tbsp rapeseed oil
- The juice of 1 lemon
- Chilli flakes

PREPARATION

1. Heat the rapeseed oil in a frying pan. Stir fry the leeks until soft. Season with salt.
2. Add in the coriander, garlic, fennel and chilli flakes.
3. After a couple of minutes, add in the spinach. Keep cooking everything on low heat until the spinach has wilted. Set aside.
4. Add extra oil into the pan and crack in the eggs. Cook until well fried.
5. Stir the yoghurt in the spinach mix. Transfer to your serving plates and top with the fried egg.
6. Season with the lemon juice, salt, black pepper and chilli flakes.

BACON & AVOCADO FRITTATA

DIFFICULTY: EASY ¦ CALORIES: 467 ¦ SERVES: 4

CARBS: 7 G ¦ FAT: 38 G ¦ PROTEIN: 22 G

INGREDIENTS

- 6 eggs, beaten
- 200 g mixed salad leaves
- 1 large avocado, halved, stoned, and cut into chunks
- 12 baby plum tomatoes, halved
- 3 tbsp olive oil
- 8 smoked bacon slices
- 2 tsp red wine vinegar
- 1 small red chilli, chopped

PREPARATION

1. Heat an ovenproof pan and fry the bacon. Chop into large pieces and set aside. Use some kitchen paper to absorb excess fat, if needed.
2. Heat 1 tbsp oil in a pan. In a bowl, break the eggs and add ½ of the bacon, and season with salt. Cook on low heat in the pan.
3. Place the avocado slices and the remaining bacon. Grill for 4-5 minutes.
4. Mix the chilli, vinegar and remaining oil and use this mixture to season the frittata.
5. Serve with the salad leaves and tomatoes.

PRAWN AND HERB OMELETTE

DIFFICULTY: EASY ¦ CALORIES: 288 ¦ SERVES: 2

CARBS: 19 G ¦ FAT: 21 G ¦ PROTEIN: 6 G

INGREDIENTS

- 4 eggs
- 250 ml milk
- 350 g prawns, cooked, peeled, chopped
- 60 g butter, diced
- 1 ½ cups mixed herbs

Lemon-Tahini Dressing

- 1 tbsp tahini
- 2 tbsp extra virgin olive oil
- 2 tbsp honey
- 2 tbsp chopped chives
- 1 lemon cut into wedges, to serve

- 2 spring onions, sliced
- 1 cucumber, sliced
- 1 fennel, sliced
- Toasted sesame seeds, to serve
- Toasted nori sheets, cut into squares

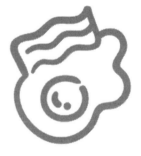

PREPARATION

1. To make the dressing, mix the tahini, olive oil, honey, lemon juice and 1 tbsp water. season with salt and stir in the chives.
2. In another bowl, mix the milk, herbs and eggs.
3. Melt ½ butter in a non-stick frying pan, then add in the egg mixture. Use a spatula to draw the cooked egg towards the centre of the pan, without breaking them up.
4. Add in half the prawn and cook until they are warmed. Transfer to a serving plate and repeat with remaining ingredients.
5. Serve topped with fennel, cucumber, spring onion, sesame seeds and nori, and the dressing.

MEXICAN EGG ROLL

DIFFICULTY: EASY ¦ CALORIES: 133 ¦ SERVES: 2

CARBS: 2 G ¦ FAT: 10 G ¦ PROTEIN: 9 G

INGREDIENTS

- 1 large egg
- 2 tbsp tomato salsa
- 1 tbsp rapeseed oil
- 1 tbsp fresh coriander

PREPARATION

1. Beat the egg along with 1 tbsp water.
2. Heat the oil in a pan and add the egg. Swirl around the base of the frying pan until you get a pancake, and cook until set.
3. Remove from heat and spread the tomato salsa over the pancake. Sprinkle with the coriander and roll it up.

Bonus: Keto-Friendly 2 Weeks Complete Diet Plan

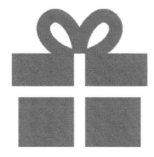

Day 1

Breakfast: Bacon & Avocado Frittata (See page 75)

Lunch: Miso Pork with Mushrooms, Beans and Chinese Broccoli

DIFFICULTY: EASY ¦ CALORIES: 287 ¦ SERVES: 4

CARBS: 19 G ¦ FAT: 10 G ¦ PROTEIN: 13 G

INGREDIENTS

- 600 g pork neck, sliced
- 100 g white miso paste
- 2 bunches Chinese broccoli
- 200 g mixed mushrooms
- 1 bunch green beans

- 2 tbsp soy sauce
- 2 tsp ginger, finely grated
- 2 tbsp brown sugar
- Toasted sesame seeds, to serve
- Fried Asian shallots, to serve

PREPARATION

1. Combine ½ of miso, the soy sauce and sugar in a large bowl, and the other half in a smaller bowl.
2. Add the pork to the big bowl and toss to coat.
3. Heat some sunflower oil in a wok and add ginger and sesame oil. Add pork and cook until caramelised, then remove from the pan.
4. Stir fry the broccoli and beans for a few minutes. Return the meat to pan for ½ minute, then cover with the reserved miso marinade.
5. Serve hot, topped with sesame seeds and fried shallots.

Dinner: Steak with Porcini Butter and Charred Onion (See page 29)

Day 2

Breakfast: Scrambled Eggs with Basil, Spinach & Tomatoes (See page 70)

Lunch: Keto Japanese Kingfish Lettuce Cups (See page 30)

Dinner: Sashimi Salmon and Pomelo Skewers

DIFFICULTY: EASY ¦ CALORIES: 149 ¦ SERVES: 4

CARBS: 11 G ¦ FAT: 13 G ¦ PROTEIN: 17 G

INGREDIENTS

- 200 g skinless sashimi-grade salmon, cut into thick slices
- 1 pomelo, cut into pieces

Coriander Root Dressing

- 1 small red chilli, chopped
- 1 ½ tbsp finely grated palm sugar
- ½ garlic clove
- 2 tbsp fish sauce
- 4 coriander roots
- The juice of 2 limes

- ½ cup Thai basil
- ½ cup coriander sprig
- Chopped roasted peanuts, to serve

PREPARATION

1. To make the coriander root dressing, pound the coriander roots and garlic with a mortar and pestle until you get a coarse paste. Transfer to a jar with a lid, add the remaining ingredients, shake well and set aside.
2. Thread the salmon and pomelo onto wooden skewers.
3. Scatter with coriander and Thai basil.
4. Drizzle with some dressing and serve with peanuts, extra chilli and the remaining coriander root dressing.

Day 3

Breakfast: Mushroom Hash with Poached Eggs (See page 69)

Lunch: Keto Pork with Ginger, Spring Onion and Eggplant

DIFFICULTY: MEDIUM ¦ CALORIES: 329 ¦ SERVES: 4

CARBS: 16 G ¦ FAT: 19 G ¦ PROTEIN: 17 G

INGREDIENTS

- 500 g pork mince
- 3 eggplant, diced
- 250 g spring onions, chopped
- 60 ml sunflower oil
- 45 ml mirin
- 30 ml soy sauce
- 60 g roasted and salted peanuts
- 15 g coriander, chopped
- 4 garlic cloves, thinly sliced
- 7 cm ginger piece, peeled
- 1 tbsp rice vinegar
- 1 tsp sesame oil
- 2 tbsp kecap manis (or sweet soy sauce)
- 1 green chilli, sliced, seeds in
- 1 tbsp sesame seeds, toasted

PREPARATION

1. Season the eggplant and transfer to a steamer.
2. Bring to the boil a saucepan full of water, then place the steamer on top and cover with the lid. Seal well to prevent the steam escaping. Steam for 12-15 minutes.
3. Heat half of the oil in a large pan and fry the onion, garlic, ginger and chilli for 5 minutes. Transfer to a small bowl.
4. Heat the remaining pan, add the pork mince and fry for 3 minutes. Add in the soy sauce, mirin, kecap manis, vinegar, and sesame oil. Season with salt if needed.
5. After 2 minutes, add in the spring onion mixture.
6. Stir in the coriander and peanuts.
7. Serve the eggplant with the remaining coriander and extra sesame seeds.

Dinner: Keto Cobb Egg Salad (See page 43)

Day 4

Breakfast: Mexican Egg Roll (See page 78)

Lunch: Broccoli Cheddar Soup (See page 67)

Dinner: Keto Stir-Fried Pork Mince with Zucchini and Mint

DIFFICULTY: EASY ¦ CALORIES: 365 ¦ SERVES: 4

CARBS: 17 G ¦ FAT: 29 G ¦ PROTEIN: 16 G

INGREDIENTS

- 500 g pork mince
- 2 zucchinis, grated
- 1 green chilli, sliced
- 2 garlic cloves, crushed
- 3 spring onions, thinly sliced
- 2 tbsp sunflower oil
- 2 ½ tbsp balsamic vinegar
- 1 tsp white sugar
- 2 ½ tbsp soy sauce
- 1/3 bunch mint leaves, to serve

PREPARATION

1. Heat the oil in a pan and fry the spring onions, chilli, and garlic.
2. Add in the pork and break it up with a wooden spoon. Cook for a few minutes, then stir in the vinegar, sugar and soy sauce. Leave to cook for a couple of minutes, or until reduced.
3. Add in the zucchini and cook for a few minutes.
4. Remove from heat and stir in half the mint.
5. Serve with scattered spring onion, the remaining mint and extra chilli (optional).

Day 5

Breakfast: Bacon & Avocado Frittata (See page 75)

Lunch: Grilled King Prawns with Celery Salad

DIFFICULTY: EASY ¦ CALORIES: 235 ¦ SERVES: 4

CARBS: 16 G ¦ FAT: 19 G ¦ PROTEIN: 16 G

INGREDIENTS

- 24 large prawns, peeled
- 3 garlic cloves, crushed
- 60 ml extra virgin oil
- 1 tsp Dijon mustard
- The juice of 1 lemon
- The zest of 1 lemon
- 1 tbsp chives, finely chopped
- 1 tbsp white wine vinegar
- 2 sticks celery
- Mint leaves
- 1 fennel bulb
- Lemon wedges, to serve

PREPARATION

1. Combine the oil, lemon zest and garlic in a bowl and brush the mixture over the prawns. Set aside for 15 minutes to marinate.
2. In another bowl, mix the mustard, oil, vinegar, and chives. Season with salt.
3. To make the celery salad, cut the celery into long strips. Slice the fennel and toss with some lemon juice. Add in the mint leaves.
4. Cook the prawns for 5 minutes, and serve with the mustard dressing and the celery salad.

Dinner: Low-Carb Pumpkin Spaghetti (See page 33)

Day 6

Breakfast: *Keto Mushroom Brunch (See page 71)*

Lunch: *Keto-friendly Cauliflower Soup (See page 66)*

Dinner: *Garlic Beef Skewers with Fennel Slaw*

DIFFICULTY: EASY ¦ CALORIES: 275 ¦ SERVES: 4

CARBS: 13 G ¦ FAT: 12 G ¦ PROTEIN: 11 G

INGREDIENTS

- 800 g beef rump
- 2 tbsp tarragon leaves, chopped
- 2 garlic cloves, crushed

- The zest of 1 lemon
- Lemon wedges, to serve

Slaw

- ¼ cabbage, sliced
- 2 tsp Dijon mustard
- 1 fennel, sliced
- 2 tbsp white wine vinegar
- ½ tsp fennel seeds, crushed

PREPARATION

1. Combine the zest, tarragon and garlic. Season with salt and set aside.
2. To make the slaw, combine all ingredients in a bowl.
3. Cut the beef into pieces and thread onto wooden or bamboo skewers.
4. Spread the tarragon mixture over the meat and cook on a chargrill over high heat for 8 minutes. Cover in foil and leave to rest for a few minutes.
5. Serve the skewers topped with the beef resting juice, tarragon mixture, slaw and extra lemon wedges.

Day 7

Breakfast: Keto Mushrooms Baked Eggs with Squashed Tomatoes (See page 72)

Lunch: Low-Carb Cauliflower Pizza (See page 38)

Dinner: Thai Pork Skewers with Chilli Dipping Sauce

DIFFICULTY: EASY ¦ CALORIES: 244 ¦ SERVES: 4

CARBS: 14 G ¦ FAT: 5 G ¦ PROTEIN: 11 G

INGREDIENTS

- 500 g pork mince
- 70 g breadcrumbs
- 60 ml rice wine vinegar
- 55 g caster sugar
- 2 small chillies
- 1 tbsp fish sauce
- 1 tsp grated ginger
- 2 tbsp green curry paste
- 2 tbsp water
- Mint and coriander leaves, to serve
- 8 wooden skewers

PREPARATION

1. Mix the pork, fish sauce, breadcrumbs, ginger and curry paste in a bowl. Cover and leave to chill for 1 hour.

2. Remove the seeds from the chillies and finely chop them. Stir over low heat with the rice wine vinegar, water, and sugar. Cook until the sugar dissolves and season with salt.

3. Shape the pork mince into 24 balls, and thread 3 onto each wooden skewer.

4. Cook for 8-10 minutes in a frying pan on medium heat.

5. Serve with mint and coriander leaves, and with the chilli dipping sauce.

Day 8

Breakfast: Keto Green Eggs (See page 74)

Lunch: Chicken Meatballs with Zucchini

DIFFICULTY: EASY ¦ CALORIES: 284 ¦ SERVES: 4

CARBS: 17 G ¦ FAT: 16 G ¦ PROTEIN: 15 G

INGREDIENTS

- 8 chicken sausages
- 2 large zucchinis
- 2 tbsp chopped basil leaves
- 2 tbsp red wine vinegar
- 2 tbsp extra virgin olive oil
- 2 tbsp pine nuts, toasted and chopped
- 30 g unsalted butter
- Extra basil, to serve

PREPARATION

1. Break the sausage with a wooden spoon and mix the meat with the basil. With wet hands, shape the meat into 16 meatballs and leave to chill and firm up for 10 minutes.
2. Cut the zucchini into long thin slices. Season with salt.
3. Heat some oil in a large frying pan and cook the meatballs for 10 minutes. Add in the vinegar, some water and butter.
4. Serve the meatball with zucchini, the sauce from the pan, extra basil and pine nuts.

Dinner: Chicken Salad Stuffed Avocado (See page 31)

Day 9

Breakfast: Mushroom Hash with Poached Eggs (See page 69)

Lunch: Keto Ginger Chicken Stir-Fry (See page 40)

Dinner: Seared Salmon with Pickled Vegetable and Watercress Salad

DIFFICULTY: EASY ¦ CALORIES: 284 ¦ SERVES: 4

CARBS: 16 G ¦ FAT: 31 G ¦ PROTEIN: 16 G

INGREDIENTS

- 4 x 160 g salmon fillets, skin on
- 180 ml red wine vinegar
- 120 g watercress
- 1 tbsp pink peppercorns
- 75 g caster sugar
- 2 tbsp buckwheat, toasted
- 1 bunch radishes, sliced
- 2 carrots, sliced
- 2 eschalots, cut into slices
- 2 tbsp fennel seeds, crushed
- 60 ml extra virgin oil

PREPARATION

1. Mix the vinegar, 180 ml water, sugar, peppercorns and fennel seeds in a saucepan. Season with salt and bring to the boil.
2. Mix the carrot, eschalot and radish in a heatproof container and pour over the vinegar mixture. Steep for at least 20 minutes.
3. In a frying pan, heat half the oil and cook the salmon until the skin is crisp. Turn and cook for another 2 minutes.
4. Drain the pickled vegetables and add in the watercress, buckwheat and oil.
5. Serve the salmon with the buckwheat salad.

Day 10

Breakfast: Keto Green Eggs (See page 74)

Lunch: Beef Tagliata with Cavolo Nero Dressing

DIFFICULTY: EASY ¦ CALORIES: 371 ¦ SERVES: 4

CARBS: 19 G ¦ FAT: 35 G ¦ PROTEIN: 21 G

INGREDIENTS

- 2 x 300 g rump steaks
- 1 garlic clove, crushed

Cavolo Nero Dressing

- 1 cavolo nero, trimmed
- 60 ml extra virgin olive oil
- 2 tbsp white balsamic vinegar
- ½ garlic clove, crushed

- 2 tbsp extra virgin olive oil
- Green salad, to serve

PREPARATION

1. To make the dressing, bring some water to the boil in a saucepan. Add in the cavolo nero and cook for ½ minutes, then refresh in ice water. Use a clean cloth to squeeze out the excess liquid. Place in a food processor with the other ingredients and process until you get a rough paste. Season with salt if needed.

2. In a small bowl, combine the oil and garlic. Season with salt and pepper and spread over the steaks.

3. Cook the meat for 4 minutes or until medium-rare. Leave to rest for 5 minutes covered in foil.

4. Serve the sliced steak with the cavolo nero dressing and some green salad.

Dinner: Keto Strawberry and Spinach Salad (See page 53)

Day 11

Breakfast: Bacon & Avocado Frittata (See page 75)

*Lunch: Keto Crispy Pork Belly Salad with Mint
and Coriander (See page 55)*

Dinner: Keto Roast Beef with Chilli Parmesan Cauliflower

DIFFICULTY: EASY ¦ CALORIES: 287 ¦ SERVES: 4

CARBS: 12 G ¦ FAT: 32 G ¦ PROTEIN: 20 G

INGREDIENTS

- 800 g beef eye fillet, tied at 3 cm intervals
- 1 small cauliflower, cut into florets
- 40 g grated parmesan
- 150 g wild rocket leaves
- 80 ml olive oil
- 2 garlic cloves, crushed
- 2 tbsp caramelised balsamic vinegar
- 1 tbsp sage leaves, chopped
- 1 long red chilli, chopped
- The juice of 1 lemon

PREPARATION

1. Preheat the oven to 200 C.
2. In a bowl, mix the garlic, 1 tbsp oil, 1 tbsp balsamic, and sage. Add the beef and toss to coat.
3. Transfer the beef on a baking tray along with the cauliflower. Drizzle with olive oil.
4. Roast for about 15 minutes. Sprinkle the cauliflower with parmesan and chilli and the remaining balsamic. Roast for further 15 minutes.
5. Cover the beef with foil and leave to rest for 5 minutes.
6. In another bowl, mix the lemon juice with the beef resting juice and some more oil. Toss the cauliflower with the rocket and drizzle the lemon and beef juice.
7. Slice the beef and serve with the cauliflower salad.

Day 12

Breakfast: Scrambled Eggs with Basil, Spinach &
Tomatoes (See page 70)

Lunch: Keto Red-Braised Pork Belly with Apple Salad (See page 44)

Dinner: Low-Carb Butter Chicken Salad

DIFFICULTY: EASY ¦ CALORIES: 196 ¦ SERVES: 4

CARBS: 9 G ¦ FAT: 17 G ¦ PROTEIN: 22 G

INGREDIENTS

- 200 g Greek yoghurt
- 250 g small tomatoes, halved
- 2 green chillies, sliced
- 1 red onion, sliced
- 1 cucumber, sliced
- 8 chicken thighs
- 50 g chopped roasted cashews
- 2 ½ tbsp tandoori paste
- 2 ½ tbsp garam masala
- 1 bunch coriander, leaves picked
- 2 tbsp chopped curry leaves (optional)
- The juice of 1 lemon
- 12 wooden or bamboo skewers

PREPARATION

1. In a baking dish, mix 70 g yoghurt, half the tandoori paste, 1 tbsp olive oil and 2/3 of the garam masala.
2. Insert the wooden or bamboo skewers through the chicken thighs. Transfer the skewers to the marinade and toss until covered. Leave to marinate for at least ½ hour.
3. Preheat the oven grill and place the skewers into it to grill for 20 minutes.
4. Meanwhile, in another bowl mix the lemon juice, onion, sugar, the remaining garam masala. Season with salt.
5. In another bowl, combine the cucumber, curry leaves, chilli and coriander.
6. In a third bowl, mix the remaining yoghurt and 1 tbsp tandoori paste. Spread this mixture across your serving plates. Add the cucumber salad.
7. Serve the skewers in your serving plates with drizzled cooking juices and shattered cashews.

Day 13

Breakfast: Keto Mushroom Brunch (See page 71)

Lunch: Satay Steak Skewers

DIFFICULTY: EASY ¦ CALORIES: 374 ¦ SERVES: 4

CARBS: 12.5 G ¦ FAT: 8 G ¦ PROTEIN: 11 G

INGREDIENTS

- 1 long red chilli, seeds removed, sliced
- 1 long green chilli, sliced
- 4 x 200 g rump steaks
- 80 ml apple cider vinegar
- 60 ml extra virgin olive oil
- 2 tbsp honey
- 140 g crunchy peanut butter
- 1 ½ tbsp Sriracha
- 1 tsp fish sauce
- The juice of 1 lime
- 1 ½ tbsp kecap manis (or your choice of sweet soy sauce)
- Coriander, to serve

PREPARATION

1. Combine the chilli and vinegar in a small bowl and set aside.
2. Preheat the chargrill pan.
3. Slice each steak into 3 strips and thread onto skewers.
4. In another small bowl, combine the honey, garlic, and oil. Brush this mixture over the skewers.
5. Cook your skewers for 2 minutes each side until cooked to your liking (we recommend medium-rare).
6. To make the satay, combine the Sriracha, kecap manis, peanut butter, fish sauce, and lime in a bowl with 60 ml of water. Stir well and season if necessary.
7. Serve the skewers with satay, the pickled chilli and some coriander.

Dinner: Keto-friendly Cauliflower Soup (See page 66)

Day 14

Breakfast: Tomato Baked Eggs (See page 73)

Lunch: Keto Chili (See page 34)

Dinner: Ras El Hanout, Yogurt and Lime Grilled Chicken

DIFFICULTY: MEDIUM ¦ CALORIES: 374 ¦ SERVES: 4

CARBS: 12 G ¦ FAT: 13 G ¦ PROTEIN: 12 G

INGREDIENTS

- 1.6 kg free-range whole chicken
- 280 g thick Greek-style yoghurt
- 30 g ras el hanout
- The juice of 1 lemon
- 2 tbsp extra virgin olive oil
- Lime wedges, to garnish

PREPARATION

1. Cut two slits in each chicken breast and leg.
2. Rub salt flakes all over the chicken.
3. In a large bowl, mix the yoghurt, ras el hanout and lemon juice. Season with salt. Add in the whole chicken and turn to coat. Leave to chill for 2 hours or overnight.
4. Preheat the oven to 180 C.
5. Remove chicken from marinade and cook for 5 cm on a hot pan.
6. Transfer to a baking tray and roast in the oven for 40 minutes.
7. Cover in foil and allow to rest for 10 minutes. Serve with lime wedges.

Day 15

Breakfast: Mexican Egg Roll (See page 78)

Lunch: Keto T-bone Steak with Asian-Style Mushrooms

DIFFICULTY: EASY ¦ CALORIES: 288 ¦ SERVES: 4

CARBS: 16 G ¦ FAT: 9 G ¦ PROTEIN: 12 G

INGREDIENTS

- 4 T-bone beef steaks
- 600 g Asian mushrooms, cut into bite-size pieces
- 60 ml rice bran oil
- 200 g sugar snaps, sliced
- 4 sticks celery, sliced

Dressing

- 60 ml mirin
- 60 ml soy sauce
- 2 tbsp rice vinegar
- 2 tsp grated ginger
- 1 red chilli, seeded, chopped
- 1 garlic clove, crushed

- ½ bunch garlic chives
- 1 cup mint leaves
- 1 cup coriander
- 2 carrots, cut into matchsticks
- ½ small red onion, sliced

PREPARATION

1. To make the dressing, mix all the ingredients until well combined.
2. To cook the steak, heat a grill pan. Brush the meat all over with oil and season with salt. Cook for 6 minutes or until medium-rare.
3. Leave the meat to rest. Meanwhile, stir fry the mushrooms in the same pan with remaining oil, until lightly charred. Season with half the dressing.
4. To make the salad, place all the herbs, carrots, celery, red onion and sugar snaps in a large bowl. Season with salt and the remaining dressing.
5. Serve the steaks with the mushrooms and extra garlic chives.

Dinner: Broccoli Cheddar Soup (See page 67)

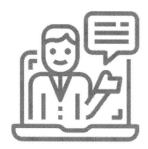

Disclaimer

This book contains opinions and ideas of the author and is meant to teach the reader informative and helpful knowledge while due care should be taken by the user in the application of the information provided. The instructions and strategies are possibly not right for every reader and there is no guarantee that they work for everyone. Using this book and implementing the information/recipes therein contained is explicitly your own responsibility and risk. This work with all its contents, does not guarantee correctness, completion, quality or correctness of the provided information. Misinformation or misprints cannot be completely eliminated.

Printed in Great Britain
by Amazon

62226081R00066